The Complete Healthy Liver Guide

A Comprehensive Guide to Understanding and Managing Liver Disease.

From Diagnosis to Treatment: Navigating the World of Liver Health

James Cloe

The complete Healthy Liver Guide: a comprehensive guide to understanding and managing liver health disease by James Cloe

Copyright© 2023 James Cloe

All rights reserved. No part of this book may be reproduced, stored in a retrieval system, or transmitted in any form or by any means, electronic, mechanical, photocopying, recording, or otherwise, without the prior written permission of the author.

Disclaimer

The information contained in this book is for educational purposes only and is not a substitute for professional medical advice, diagnosis, or treatment.

Please seek the advice of a licensed healthcare provider before making changes to your health or wellness routine. The author and publisher of this book have made every effort to ensure the accuracy and completeness of the information contained in this book. However, assume no responsibility for errors or omissions.

The information expressed in this book is solely those of the author and does not reflect the views of any organization they may be affiliated with.

Contents

INTRODUCTION 5

CHAPTER 1 7

Understanding the Liver 7

and Its Functions 7

1.1 Anatomy of the Liver 7

1.2 Functions of the Liver 8

1.3 Common Liver Diseases 9

Chapter 2 10

Common Types of Liver Diseases, Their Causes, and Symptoms 10

Hepatitis A, B, and C 10

Cirrhosis 11

Non-alcoholic Fatty Liver Disease (NAFLD) 12

Hemochromatosis 14

CHAPTER 3 16

Diagnosis and Testing for Liver Disease 16

Physical Exam 16

Blood Tests 17

Imaging Tests 17

Biopsy 17

FibroScan 18

CHAPTER 4 19

Medical Treatments for Liver Diseases: Medication and Lifestyle Changes..19

    Medication 19

    Lifestyle Changes..20

  CHAPTER 5 27

Alternative Therapies for Liver Health......................................27

    Dietary Changes 27

  CHAPTER 6 30

Liver Protecting Compounds...30

    Curcumin..30

    Anthocyanins 32

    Magnesium 33

    Apigenin 34

  CHAPTER 7 36

Coping with Liver Disease: Emotional Support.......................36

    Emotional Support 36

  CHAPTER 8 40

Prevention of Liver Disease through Healthy Habits and Vaccination..40

  CHAPTER 9 43

Managing Symptoms, Working with Healthcare Providers, and Staying Informed on the Latest Treatments...........................43

    Managing Symptoms 43

    Working with Healthcare Providers................................44

    Staying informed on the latest treatments 45

INTRODUCTION

One of the most stressful occurrences in a person's life is receiving a critical liver illness diagnosis. Such a diagnosis raises a lot of questions. Will my symptoms deteriorate further? What will the procedures entail? How will my life change, you ask? Am I going to pass away? "Am I able to improve?" The answers to these questions are frequently ambiguous, but the knowledge that is accessible might help patients prepare. This is why managing information is crucial to living with liver illness.

The same trend won't be followed by everyone. How a person responds to an illness – and information about the condition – on a daily basis will depend on their particular personality. Information requirements for patients could alter over time.

In the United States today, millions of Americans suffer from a chronic conditions like diabetes, heart disease, or irritable bowel syndrome. Despite the recent advancements in modern medicine, clinicians still frequently don't fully understand chronic illness. It is especially true with the liver that science has not fully understood the body's capacities and functioning.

People are aware of other organs in their bodies, such as the colon or the heart, but most people don't give their livers much thought. They're not required to. The remarkable capacities of the liver are not easily visible unless there is a severe breakdown in functioning. The liver works diligently to ensure that people remain healthy, even if its critical function in preserving health may not be recognized.

CHAPTER 1

Understanding the Liver and Its Functions

The liver is one of the most important organs in the human body. It plays a critical role in many of the body's functions and processes, making it essential to good health. In this chapter, we'll explore the anatomy of the liver and the vital functions it performs.

1.1 Anatomy of the Liver

The liver is a large, reddish-brown organ that sits just below the ribcage on the right side of the abdomen. It 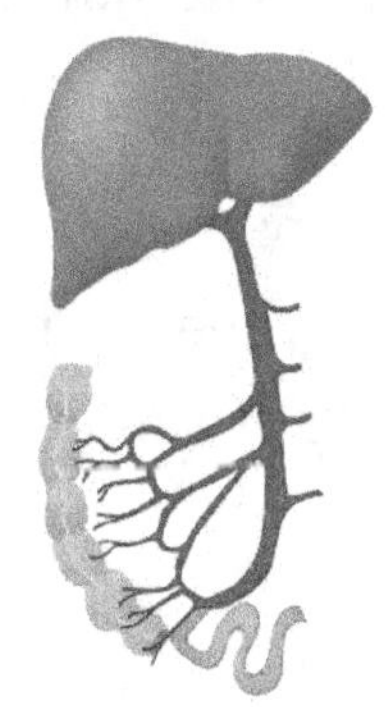 is divided into two main lobes, which are connected by a narrow band of tissue called the liver ligament. The liver weighs about 3 pounds and is shaped like a wedge.

1.2 Functions of the Liver

The liver is involved in a wide range of essential functions in the body, including:

Metabolism: The liver helps regulate the metabolism of carbohydrates, fats, and proteins. It stores glucose in the form of glycogen and releases it into the bloodstream when necessary.

Detoxification: The liver removes toxins and waste products from the bloodstream, including drugs, alcohol, and other harmful substances.

Bile production: The liver produces bile, which is necessary for the digestion and absorption of fats and fat-soluble vitamins.

Blood clotting: The liver plays a key role in the blood-clotting process, producing and storing substances that help the blood to clot.

Vitamin and mineral storage: The liver stores important vitamins and minerals, including vitamin A, vitamin D, and iron.

Immune system regulation: The liver helps regulate the immune system by producing immune cells and removing old or damaged immune cells from the bloodstream.

These are just a few of the many functions of the liver. As you can see, the liver is a crucial organ in the human body, and it's essential to take good care of it to ensure optimal health.

1.3 Common Liver Diseases

Despite its importance, the liver can be vulnerable to a range of diseases, including viral hepatitis, cirrhosis, liver cancer, and non-alcoholic fatty liver disease. In the following chapters, we'll explore these and other liver diseases in greater detail, including their causes, symptoms, and treatments.

In conclusion, the liver is a complex and essential organ that plays a vital role in the body. By understanding its anatomy and functions, you can take better care of your liver and maintain good health.

Chapter 2

Common Types of Liver Diseases, Their Causes, and Symptoms

The liver is a vital organ in the body, responsible for many important functions such as filtering toxins from the blood, producing bile for digestion, and regulating hormones. However, despite its importance, the liver is vulnerable to a range of diseases and conditions that can negatively impact its health. In this chapter, we will explore some of the most common types of liver diseases, their causes, and symptoms.

Hepatitis A, B, and C

Hepatitis refers to inflammation of the liver and is caused by a viral infection. There are three main types of viral hepatitis: Hepatitis A, B, and C.

Hepatitis A is typically spread through contaminated food or water and is less severe than other forms of hepatitis. Symptoms may include fatigue, jaundice, abdominal pain, and loss of appetite.

Hepatitis B is transmitted through contaminated blood and bodily fluids, and can lead to serious liver damage if left untreated. Symptoms can range from mild to severe, including fatigue, jaundice, dark urine, and joint pain.

Hepatitis C is spread through contaminated blood and is often asymptomatic, meaning that people may be infected without knowing it. However, it can lead to serious liver damage if left untreated. Symptoms may include fatigue, jaundice, abdominal pain, and joint pain.

Cirrhosis

Cirrhosis is a condition that occurs when the liver is damaged and scarred over time. It is most often caused by long-term alcohol abuse, but can also be caused by other factors such as hepatitis, non-alcoholic fatty liver disease, and hereditary diseases. Symptoms may include fatigue, jaundice, abdominal swelling, and confusion.

Non-alcoholic Fatty Liver Disease (NAFLD)

Non-alcoholic fatty liver disease refers to a build-up of fat in the liver that is not caused by alcohol consumption. It is often associated with obesity, high cholesterol, and high blood pressure. Symptoms may include fatigue, abdominal pain, and elevated liver enzymes on blood tests.

Non-alcoholic steatohepatitis (NASH), which is caused by the buildup of fat in the liver, can result in inflammation and scarring as well as cirrhosis, liver failure, and even liver cancer. Up to 25% of the world's population may be affected by NAFLD, which is now regarded as the most prevalent liver disease in affluent nations.

Although the precise origin of NAFLD is not fully understood, it is thought to be related to a number of variables, such as obesity, insulin resistance, high cholesterol, and excessive triglycerides. The risk of developing NAFLD is also higher in people with sedentary lifestyles, high-sugar diets, and poor fat intake.

Many people may not even be aware they have NAFLD because the symptoms are frequently mild. Fatigue, abdominal pain, and a general sense of discomfort in the upper right abdomen are, however, some typical symptoms. In some situations, people with NAFLD may also develop fluid buildup in the belly and yellowing of the skin and eyes (jaundice) (ascites).

NAFLD is often diagnosed using a combination of a medical history, physical examination, and imaging tests like an MRI or ultrasound. Blood tests may also be used to assess liver health and look for high liver enzyme concentrations, which may indicate liver disease.

A balanced diet reduced in sugar and harmful fats, frequent exercise, and weight loss are common components of NAFLD treatment. Additionally, medications may be recommended to control underlying diseases including diabetes and high cholesterol. Liver transplantation can be required in extreme situations.

If you are exhibiting any NAFLD symptoms, you should consult a doctor right away because prompt treatment can significantly improve your prognosis and stop the disease's progression. Maintaining a healthy lifestyle and making necessary lifestyle modifications are essential for controlling NAFLD and lowering the risk of more severe liver problems.

Find below a link to few health products I would greatly recommend to you. A lot of people have testified of their effectiveness against fatty liver disease.

1. Fatty liver remedy

2. Reverse Your Fatty Liver

3. Liver Support

Hemochromatosis

Hemochromatosis is a genetic condition that causes the body to absorb and store too much iron. This can lead to liver damage and cirrhosis over time. Symptoms may include joint pain, fatigue, and abdominal pain.

It is important to understand that liver disease can be silent and not have any obvious symptoms until the disease is well advanced. Regular check-ups and monitoring of liver function through blood tests can help detect liver disease early and improve the chances of successful treatment.

In conclusion, liver diseases can range from mild to severe, and can be caused by viral infections, alcohol consumption, obesity, genetics, and other factors. Understanding the common types of liver diseases, their causes, and symptoms is crucial for maintaining good liver health and seeking prompt treatment if necessary.

CHAPTER 3

Diagnosis and Testing for Liver Disease

Diagnosing liver disease early is crucial for successful treatment and management. In this chapter, we will explore the various tests and procedures used to diagnose liver disease, and what to expect during the diagnostic process.

Physical Exam

The first step in diagnosing liver disease is a physical exam. During this exam, your doctor will look for signs of liver disease, such as jaundice (yellowing of the skin and eyes), abdominal swelling, and a tender liver. Your doctor may also ask about your symptoms, medical history, and risk factors for liver disease.

Blood Tests

Blood tests are a common and important part of the diagnostic process for liver disease. Blood tests can detect elevated levels of liver enzymes, which can indicate liver damage, or abnormal levels of certain chemicals in the blood, such as bilirubin or prothrombin time. Blood tests can also be used to detect the presence of viral hepatitis or other liver diseases.

Imaging Tests

Imaging tests such as ultrasound, CT scan, or MRI can be used to view the liver and determine if there is any damage or abnormality. These tests can also help to identify the underlying cause of liver disease, such as fatty liver disease or cirrhosis.

Biopsy

A biopsy is a procedure in which a small piece of liver tissue is removed and examined under a microscope to determine the cause and extent of liver damage. A biopsy can also be used to determine the stage of liver disease and determine the best course of treatment.

FibroScan

FibroScan is a non-invasive test that uses ultrasound technology to assess the stiffness of the liver and determine the presence of liver disease. This test is especially useful for detecting early stages of liver fibrosis or cirrhosis.

It is important to understand that liver disease can be difficult to diagnose, and a combination of tests may be needed to reach a diagnosis. It is also important to work closely with your doctor to determine the best course of action, and to receive prompt treatment if necessary.

In conclusion, the diagnostic process for liver disease involves a physical exam, blood tests, imaging tests, biopsy, and fibroscan. Early detection is crucial for successful treatment and management, and it is important to work closely with your doctor to determine the best course of action.

CHAPTER 4

Medical Treatments for Liver Diseases: Medication and Lifestyle Changes

When it comes to treating liver disease, there is no one-size-fits-all solution. The appropriate treatment depends on the underlying cause of the liver disease and the stage of the disease. In this chapter, we will discuss the different medical treatments available for liver diseases, including medication and lifestyle changes.

Medication

Medications are often used to treat liver diseases by reducing inflammation, preventing the virus from replicating, or managing symptoms. The specific medication used will depend on the type of liver disease and the stage of the disease. Some common medications used to treat liver diseases include:

Interferon: Used to treat Hepatitis B and C. Interferon works by reducing the amount of virus in the blood.

Antiviral medications: Antiviral medications are used to treat Hepatitis B and C and work by inhibiting the replication of the virus.

Antifibrotic medications: Antifibrotic medications are used to treat cirrhosis and work by slowing down the progression of fibrosis in the liver.

Antioxidants: Antioxidants such as Vitamin E and N-acetyl cysteine can help reduce oxidative stress in the liver and improve liver function.

It's important to note that while medications can help manage liver disease, they cannot cure it. Therefore, it's crucial to work closely with your doctor to determine the best course of treatment for your specific condition.

Lifestyle Changes

In addition to medication, lifestyle changes can play a significant role in managing liver disease and improving liver health. Some important lifestyle changes that can help improve liver health include:

Reducing alcohol consumption: Alcohol consumption can significantly damage the liver, so it's crucial to limit alcohol consumption or avoid it altogether.

The liver, which is in charge of eliminating toxins from the body, is poisonous to alcohol. The liver gets overburdened and unable to cope when a person consumes excessive amounts of alcohol. This may harm the liver's cells over time, eventually resulting in cirrhosis. A dangerous disorder called cirrhosis can result in the liver becoming damaged and functioning less efficiently. Liver failure and other severe problems, such liver cancer, may result from this.

Another deadly liver disease that can be brought on by alcohol is hepatitis. Hepatitis can develop as a result of liver inflammation brought on by alcohol. Serious liver damage from this can result in cirrhosis and liver failure. The dangerous and frequently fatal disorder known as liver cancer is also significantly increased by alcohol.

Alcohol use is more strongly linked to liver damage among heavy and frequent drinkers. This is due to the liver's inability to keep up with demands, which over time causes catastrophic damage. People who are already at risk, such as those with a family history of liver disease or those who have certain liver disorders, are also more likely to develop liver disease as a result of alcohol.

The risk of liver disease brought on by alcohol can be decreased in a number of ways. The first step is to consume less alcohol. This entails consuming alcohol in moderation, such as one drink per day for women and two drinks per day for men. Additionally, it's vital to mix up your alcohol use rather than sticking to just one kind, as this can lower your risk of developing liver disease.

The 7-day Drink less Mind program has guaranteed results of helping people get off the drinking too much treadmill.

Maintaining a healthy diet: A healthy diet that is low in fat and high in fiber can help improve liver function and reduce the risk of liver disease.

Reduced risk of obesity and metabolic syndrome is one of the key ways that a nutritious diet can help prevent liver disease. Because they put a heavy burden on the liver and may result in inflammation, scarring, and other damage, these conditions are known to raise the risk of developing liver disease. A diet high in fresh produce, lean protein, whole grains, and healthy fats can help lower the risk of many diseases and maintain the function of the liver.

Keeping toxins and other dangerous chemicals in check in the diet is another crucial aspect of preventing liver disease. This entails consuming less alcohol, staying away from coffee with a high caffeine content, and cutting back on processed and junk food. Antioxidants and other healthy substances found in foods can help reduce inflammation and safeguard the liver from harm.

A balanced diet can be especially helpful for those who already have liver disease. This is due to the fact that a balanced diet can assist to improve the general health of the liver and to lessen the symptoms of liver disease. High-fiber, vitamin- and mineral-rich diets can lower the risk of liver disease and enhance the health of people who already have liver issues.

Exercising regularly: Regular exercise can help reduce oxidative stress and improve liver function. Regular exercise is important for maintaining good liver health, as well as overall physical and mental well-being. Gentle exercises, such as walking, yoga, and swimming, are great for people with liver disease, as they can help improve circulation, boost energy levels, and reduce stress.

However, it's important to talk to your doctor before starting an exercise program, as some forms of liver disease can cause fatigue and muscle weakness. Your doctor can help you determine what type and amount of exercise is appropriate for your individual needs.

Maintaining a healthy weight:

Weight has a significant impact on liver disease since it can affect both the progression and management of pre-existing liver illnesses as well as the chance of developing new liver issues.

One of the major risk factors for liver disease is being obese. The extra fat that builds up in the body makes the liver work harder, which can result in inflammation and liver damage. This causes the liver to scar, or create hepatic fibrosis, which can progress to cirrhosis and liver failure.

The chance of developing fatty liver disease, a disorder in which fat builds up in the liver, is also increased by weight gain. Inflammation, liver injury, and ultimately liver scarring can result from this. Additionally, having a large waistline or being obese raises the possibility of getting hepatitis, liver cancer, and bile duct illnesses, which are all conditions of the liver.

The health of the liver, however, can benefit from weight loss. The stress on the liver can be lessened, and liver function can be improved, by reducing the amount of fat that is stored there. As a result, there is a lower chance of acquiring liver disease and a slower rate of deterioration of current liver problems.

I found this weight loosing product very good and would gladly recommend.

Use this link to get one: Puradrop

Managing stress: Chronic stress can increase oxidative stress and negatively impact liver function, so it's important to find ways to manage stress, such as meditation, yoga, or exercise.

Get adequate sleep: Sleep plays a crucial role in liver health, and a lack of sleep has been linked to an increased risk of liver disease. Aim to get at least 7-8 hours of sleep per night.

In conclusion, liver disease is a complex condition that requires a combination of medical treatment and lifestyle changes to manage effectively. Medications can help manage symptoms and reduce the progression of the disease, while lifestyle changes can help improve liver health and reduce the risk of liver disease. It's important to work closely with your doctor to determine the best course of treatment for your specific condition.

CHAPTER 5

Alternative Therapies for Liver Health

In addition to conventional medical treatments, there are a number of alternative therapies that can help improve liver health and function. These therapies include dietary changes, herbal remedies, and lifestyle modifications. Let's take a closer look at each of these therapies and how they can help support liver health.

Dietary Changes

One of the most important steps you can take to improve liver health is to adopt a healthy diet. A diet that is high in fiber, lean protein, and antioxidants can help protect the liver and reduce the risk of liver disease. Some of the best foods for liver health include:

Leafy green vegetables, such as spinach and kale, which are high in antioxidants and help reduce inflammation.

Cruciferous vegetables, such as broccoli and cauliflower, which have been shown to have liver-protective effects.

Berries, such as blueberries, raspberries, and strawberries, which are high in antioxidants and can help reduce inflammation.

Nuts and seeds, such as almonds, walnuts, and flaxseeds, which are high in fiber and healthy fats.

It is also important to limit your consumption of foods that can be harmful to the liver, such as processed foods, high-fat foods, and alcohol.

Herbal Remedies

There are a number of herbs that have been traditionally used to support liver health and function. Some of the most commonly used herbs include:

Milk thistle, which is thought to protect the liver from toxins and support liver cell regeneration. Studies has as well shown that milk thistle can repair damaged liver cells. Milk thistle contains silymarin, a flavonoid which provides the liver with protection against many toxins.

Milk thistle is a really great product for liver health. And if you would want one, get it here.

Dandelion root, which is known for its liver-detoxifying effects and is commonly used to support liver function.

Turmeric: it is a powerful antioxidant that has anti-inflammatory properties and may help protect the liver from damage.

Artichoke: it has been shown to improve liver function and reduce symptoms of liver disease.

It is important to remember that while herbal remedies can be helpful, they can also interact with other medications you may be taking. Therefore, it is always best to consult with a healthcare professional before taking any new herbs or supplements.

In conclusion, there are a number of alternative therapies that can help support liver health and function. Adopting a healthy diet, using herbal remedies, and making lifestyle modifications can all help protect the liver and reduce the risk of liver disease. However, it is important to consult with a healthcare professional before making any significant changes to your diet or lifestyle, and to seek prompt medical attention if you have symptoms of liver disease.

CHAPTER 6

Liver Protecting Compounds

Curcumin

Curcumin is a substance found in the spice turmeric, which is frequently used in food and conventional medicine. The active component of turmeric, curcumin, has been the focus of numerous studies because of its possible health advantages. Curcumin has showed promise in a number of areas, including liver health.

According to studies, curcumin may aid in the liver's general health and damage prevention. It has been discovered that curcumin possesses antioxidant capabilities that aid in scavenging dangerous free radicals that can affect the liver. Additionally, since liver inflammation is a prominent cause of liver damage, it might aid in reducing liver inflammation.

Curcumin can also help the liver function by enhancing its capacity to eliminate toxic chemicals. Curcumin has been shown in studies to increase the activity of particular enzymes involved in detoxification, making it simpler for the liver to eliminate toxins from the body. This may lessen the strain on the liver and help it to work more efficiently.

Curcumin has also been demonstrated to have potential advantages in the treatment of cirrhosis and fatty liver disease, among other liver conditions. Curcumin has been shown to lessen liver inflammation and fatty liver disease in animal experiments. By lowering oxidative stress and inflammation, it may also assist to stop the advancement of cirrhosis.

Curcumin's potential health advantages for the liver seem encouraging. Curcumin can be found in turmeric and pills, and including it in your diet through these means may promote liver function, however more research is required to completely understand its effects. However, it's crucial to speak with a doctor before beginning any new supplement program, especially if you already have liver issues.

Anthocyanins

The red, blue, and purple hues of fruits and vegetables come from a class of flavonoids called anthocyanins. Recent research suggests that these substances might benefit liver health.

Anthocyanins' advantages for the liver include:

- Anthocyanins have been found to have potent antioxidant capabilities that aid in scavenging dangerous free radicals and shielding the liver from oxidative stress.
- Anthocyanins have also been found to have anti-inflammatory properties that may aid to protect the liver from harm. Inflammation has been linked to the development of liver disease.
- Reduction of oxidative stress and inflammation that can cause liver damage: Studies have indicated that anthocyanins can assist to protect the liver against hazardous substances, including medicines and chemicals.

Although the research on anthocyanins' health advantages for liver function is encouraging, it is crucial to remember that further research is required to completely understand their effects and set guidelines for ideal intake.

Blackberries, blueberries, cherries, raspberries, red grapes, blackcurrants, and red onions are a few examples of foods that contain anthocyanins. To possibly benefit from anthocyanins' benefits for liver health, it is advised to include a range of these foods in your diet.

Magnesium

Magnesium is a necessary mineral that is required for sustaining healthy liver function. The liver performs numerous crucial tasks such creating bile, removing toxins from the blood, and controlling blood sugar and cholesterol levels. A sufficient magnesium intake can support the liver's optimal performance.

- Magnesium supports the liver's detoxification process by turning on enzymes that break down poisons and toxic chemicals. As a result, the liver isn't put under as much stress and can work more effectively.
- Reduces Inflammation: Due to its anti-inflammatory qualities, magnesium can aid in reducing liver inflammation. Magnesium is a crucial component for liver health since chronic liver inflammation can result in a number of liver disorders.
- Magnesium aids in regulating glucose metabolism, which is critical for the functioning of the liver. Adequate magnesium consumption can maintain proper glucose metabolism and

lower the risk of liver disease. The liver helps manage the body's glucose levels.

- Supports Bile Production: Bile, a substance that aids in the digestion of fats and the absorption of fat-soluble vitamins, is produced in part by magnesium. The liver can create enough bile to sustain healthy digestion and liver function with the aid of an adequate magnesium intake.

One more time, I found you a highly recommended magnesium nutrient supplement I use at home.

[Get it here!](#)

Apigenin

Plants including chamomile, parsley, and celery are rich sources of the flavonoid apigenin which is well known for its anti-inflammatory, antioxidant, and anti-carcinogenic qualities. Apigenin may benefit the health of the liver, according to recent studies.

The ability of apigenin to defend against oxidative stress is one of the substance's key advantages for the liver. Antioxidants like apigenin assist in scavenging free radicals that might injure the liver's cells and are always present in the body. Apigenin can do this to protect the liver and enhance liver function in general.

Reduced inflammation is another way that apigenin might help the liver. Apigenin has been found to have anti-inflammatory actions in both animal and human research. Chronic inflammation is a significant contributor to the onset of liver illnesses such fatty liver disease.

Apigenin has also demonstrated to be effective against liver cancer in addition to its anti-inflammatory and antioxidant characteristics. According to research, apigenin can stop the growth of liver cancer cells and cause cell death. This is probably as a result of its capacity to engage with particular molecular pathways related to cancer.

Overall, the research indicates that by lowering oxidative stress, inflammation, and cancer risk, apigenin can play a significant role in preserving liver health. More research is necessary to completely comprehend the effects of apigenin on the liver and to establish the best dosage and timeframe for supplementation, it is vital to mention.

To completely comprehend apigenin's effects on the liver and to establish the ideal dosage and supplementation period, more research is nonetheless required.

CHAPTER 7

Coping with Liver Disease: Emotional Support

Living with liver disease can be a challenging experience, but it is possible to maintain a good quality of life with the right support, diet, and exercise. In this chapter, we will explore some effective strategies for coping with liver disease, including emotional support, diet, and exercise.

Emotional Support

Living with liver disease can be emotionally challenging, and it's important to have a supportive network of family and friends to help you through the ups and downs. Joining a support group for people with liver disease can also be a valuable source of comfort, advice, and encouragement. Talking to a mental health professional, such as a counsellor or therapist, can also help you manage the emotional impact of liver disease and develop healthy coping strategies.

Denial, anger, bargaining, sadness, and acceptance are the five general stages of adjustment that patients may go through when dealing with a significant liver condition. However, they have since shown to be applicable to patients with chronic liver disorders or for whom recovery is conceivable but questionable. Elisabeth Kübler-Ross first used these stages to explain the process of coming to grips with a fatal diagnosis in her seminal book, On Death and Dying.

Your reaction to learning that you have liver disease may be tough to manage emotionally. You can feel angry, overburdened, and concerned about the future. You might wish to talk to folks close to you as the news begins to set in and express your feelings, worries, and inquiries.

Sharing your worries and expressing how you're feeling might reassure you and support you in managing your diagnosis both now and in the future. Furthermore, telling your loved ones about your disease will enable them to support you and help you with any necessary lifestyle adjustments.

It is advised that you learn as much as you can about your condition from reliable sources, give it some thought, and take action.

It is crucial to have daily assistance and attention. But it's not always simple to discuss the illness with your loved ones. When learning of a disease condition, every person responds differently. It is crucial to base your explanation on the unique personality of each person. In fact, while some people choose to learn practical skills, others seek scholarly information to better comprehend the disease.

Making the decision to inform someone can be challenging and frequently private. You might want to pause and consider your actions before spreading the news too widely. Due to the stigma attached to certain liver disorders, such as viral hepatitis and alcohol-related liver disease, some people may not feel comfortable discussing their diagnosis.

Preconceived notions could prevent you from getting the support you'd like. Consider the potential response. If you begin to feel exposed after receiving your diagnosis, don't forget to take precautions. Make sure you're sure the person you want to inform will respect you and your condition and be supportive of you.

It might also be appealing to you to ask for help from random people. Being reserved and just discussing your situation in an anonymous way is not shameful. Seeking support can truly make you feel like you're not on your own, whether it be in person at a nearby support group, over the phone on a helpline, or speaking with folks online via a forum.

Additionally, using the internet for help has the advantage that, whenever you log on, someone is generally available for a chat. On Facebook and on specialized websites like Health Unlocked, there are a variety of particular online support groups (UK). For those who feel alone because of their liver illness, these online networks can frequently be a lifeline.

CHAPTER 8

Prevention of Liver Disease through Healthy Habits and Vaccination

Liver disease is a serious condition that can have long-term impacts on health and quality of life. Fortunately, many liver diseases can be prevented or managed through lifestyle changes and vaccinations. In this chapter, we will explore some of the key strategies for preventing liver disease through healthy habits and vaccination.

Healthy Habits

Healthy habits play a critical role in maintaining liver health and preventing liver disease. Some of the key habits that can help prevent liver disease include:

Maintaining a healthy weight: Excess body weight, especially around the midsection, can increase the risk of liver disease, especially non-alcoholic fatty liver disease. Eating a balanced diet, engaging in regular physical activity, and reducing sugar and processed food intake can help maintain a healthy weight.

Limiting alcohol consumption: Excessive alcohol consumption is one of the leading causes of liver disease, and can lead to cirrhosis and liver failure. Limiting alcohol intake to the recommended daily limits of no more than 2 drinks for men and 1 drink for women can help protect the liver.

Avoiding exposure to toxins: Certain toxins, such as excessive amounts of acetaminophen (found in some pain relievers), can be harmful to the liver. Limiting exposure to these toxins and following product label instructions can help protect the liver.

Practicing safe sex: Sexually transmitted infections such as hepatitis B and C can cause liver damage and increase the risk of liver disease. Practicing safe sex and getting vaccinated against Hepatitis B can help protect against sexually transmitted infections.

Vaccination

Vaccination is an effective and safe way to prevent the spread of certain viral infections that can lead to liver disease. There are two main types of vaccines that can help prevent liver disease:

Hepatitis A vaccine: The Hepatitis A vaccine can protect against the Hepatitis A virus, which is spread through contaminated food or water. This vaccine is typically recommended for people who are at high risk of infection, such as travellers to certain countries or those who work in close contact with contaminated food or water.

Hepatitis B vaccine: The Hepatitis B vaccine can protect against the Hepatitis B virus, which is spread through contaminated blood and bodily fluids. This vaccine is recommended for all new-borns and at-risk individuals, such as health care workers and people who have multiple sexual partners.

In conclusion, liver disease can be prevented through healthy habits and vaccination. By maintaining a healthy weight, limiting alcohol consumption, avoiding exposure to toxins, and getting vaccinated, people can reduce their risk of liver disease and maintain good liver health. Regular check-ups and monitoring of liver function through blood tests can also help detect liver disease early and improve the chances of successful treatment.

CHAPTER 9

Managing Symptoms, Working with Healthcare Providers, and Staying Informed on the Latest Treatments

Being diagnosed with liver disease can be overwhelming and frightening. However, with the right support and care, it is possible to manage symptoms, maintain good health, and live a fulfilling life. In this chapter, we will explore various strategies for living with liver disease, including managing symptoms, working with healthcare providers, and staying informed on the latest treatments.

Managing Symptoms

Managing symptoms of liver disease is a crucial part of maintaining good health and quality of life. Some common symptoms of liver disease include fatigue, abdominal pain, jaundice, and confusion. Here are some tips for managing these symptoms:

Eat a healthy, balanced diet: A healthy diet can help manage symptoms and improve overall health.

Working with Healthcare Providers

Working with a healthcare provider is essential for managing liver disease. Here are some tips for working effectively with your healthcare provider:

Find a specialist: Find a healthcare provider who specializes in liver disease to ensure that you receive the best possible care.

Communicate openly and honestly: It is important to communicate openly and honestly with your healthcare provider about your symptoms and concerns.

Keep track of your symptoms and medical history: Keeping a record of your symptoms and medical history can help your healthcare provider diagnose and treat liver disease more effectively.

Ask questions and seek clarification: Don't be afraid to ask questions and seek clarification from your healthcare provider to ensure that you fully understand your condition and treatment options.

Staying informed on the latest treatments

Staying informed on the latest treatments for liver disease is essential for maintaining good health and quality of life. Here are some tips for staying informed on the latest treatments:

Read reputable medical journals and websites: Keep up to date on the latest developments in liver disease research and treatment by reading reputable medical journals and websites.

Attend support groups: Attend support groups to connect with others living with liver disease and stay informed on the latest treatments and advancements.

Ask your healthcare provider: Ask your healthcare provider about the latest treatments and advancements in liver disease to stay informed.

In conclusion, living with liver disease can be challenging, but with the right support and care, it is possible to manage symptoms, maintain good health, and live a fulfilling life. By managing symptoms, working effectively with healthcare providers, and staying informed on the latest treatments, people with liver disease can take control of their health and live their best lives.

1. <u>Fatty liver remedy</u>
2. <u>Reverse Your Fatty Liver</u>
3. <u>Liver Support</u>
4. <u>Weight loss product: **Puradrop**</u>
5. <u>The 7-day Drink less Mind program has guaranteed results of helping people get off the drinking too much treadmill.</u>
6. <u>Milk thistle</u>
7. <u>Magnesium nutrient supplement</u>

The links above would help you get easy access to few of the products I recommended in this book to promoting the health of your liver.

I hope you found the content of this ebook, including the recommended products very helpful.

If you did, don't forget to recommend to your family and friends and also leave behind a review to help us improve.